Distribution, publication, and copying in any form are prohibited and subject to damages.

TEN HYPNOSES

Copying, publishing, and sharing with third parties are only permitted with the written consent of the author. Please observe the notes on copyright and usage.

Distribution, publication, and copying in any form are prohibited and subject to damages.

Copying, publishing, and sharing with third parties are only permitted with the written consent of the author. Please observe the notes on copyright and usage.

Distribution, publication, and copying in any form are prohibited and subject to damages.

Ingo Michael Simon

TEN HYPNOSES

45
FEAR OF THE DARK

Copying, publishing, and sharing with third parties are only permitted with the written consent of the author. Please observe the notes on copyright and usage.

Distribution, publication, and copying in any form are prohibited and subject to damages.

© 2024 Ingo Michael Simon
All rights reserved.
Independently published
www.ingosimon.com

Important Notes for Urgent Attention:

The contents of this book are based on the practical experiences of the author with hypnosis applications and psychotherapy in a trance state. Although the author has strived for the utmost care, errors or misunderstandings in the presentation cannot be completely excluded. Therapeutic work with people and the application of hypnosis are solely the responsibility of the hypnotist. It cannot be ruled out that parts of this book may be misunderstood or that the application of a presented procedure may cause an undesirable reaction in the client. The author also assumes no co-responsibility if work with a client is carried out with reference to the statements in this book.

The Author:

Ingo Michael Simon studied psychology and education and is a hypnotherapist with practices in southwestern Germany and Switzerland. With the help of hypnosis-supported psychotherapy, he primarily treats people with persistent psychological conditions. His practice focuses on anxiety disorders, pathological compulsions, and psychosomatic illnesses. His therapeutic offerings mainly include classical and modern hypnosis applications and the dreamland therapy he developed himself.

Copying, publishing, and sharing with third parties are only permitted with the written consent of the author. Please observe the notes on copyright and usage.

Distribution, publication, and copying in any form are prohibited and subject to damages.

INTRODUCTION	6
COPYRIGHT AND USAGE	8
HYPNOSIS 1	10
HYPNOSIS 2	15
HYPNOSIS 3	20
HYPNOSIS 4	25
HYPNOSIS 5	30
HYPNOSIS 6	35
HYPNOSIS 7	39
HYPNOSIS 8	44
HYPNOSIS 9	50
HYPNOSIS 10	56
ALL TITLES IN THE SERIES	61

Copying, publishing, and sharing with third parties are only permitted with the written consent of the author. Please observe the notes on copyright and usage.

Introduction

The series "Ten Hypnoses" is very well known in Germany, Austria, and Switzerland as a collection of texts for therapeutic work and is used by numerous psychotherapeutic practices, doctors, therapists, coaches, and other helping professionals. I am pleased to now be able to offer these texts in other countries as well.

Most therapists have their own methods for inducing and deepening trance as well as for exiting trance. Therefore, I have focused on the main part of the hypnosis. The texts in this book can be integrated as the main part into any hypnosis process. The texts in this collection use various hypnosis techniques. I will not explain these in detail, as I assume that users have the appropriate training. It is also not necessary to understand the exact structure or functioning of the different parts. The texts can simply be read aloud, and they will have their effect.

Decide for yourself which text best suits your client or patient at any given time. You can also combine passages from different texts. It is not about using all ten hypnoses in sequence. It is a selection of possibilities.

I want to emphasize that books cannot replace therapy. Psychotherapy or other therapeutic treatments involve much more. A careful diagnosis is the necessary basis for deciding on the use of methods, including whether hypnosis or one of my texts should be used. Even in this case, preparatory discussions, follow-up discussions during the session, and of course, a therapeutic concept for the sequence of sessions and the content approaches are essential parts of therapy. This cannot and should not be achieved with a collection of texts.

In any case, I wish you much success in your work and I am pleased if my text templates can contribute in a small way.

Ingo Michael Simon

Copyright and Usage

Copying, publishing, and sharing with third parties is prohibited and only permitted with the written consent of the author. Please observe the following copyright and usage guidelines.

This work has been carefully crafted and created to the best of the author's knowledge and personal experience. It comprises text templates and application guidelines for professional hypnosis sessions. The author is a licensed psychotherapist with extensive experience in psychotherapy, coaching, and personal training using hypnotic techniques and methods. Nevertheless, the author and the publisher assume no liability for the accuracy of information, instructions, and advice, nor for any typographical errors. The author and publisher accept no responsibility or liability for the application of these texts and recommendations with clients or patients, nor for any potential consequences or unexpected reactions. It is expressly noted that the application of therapeutic and advisory techniques and formulations lies solely and entirely within the responsibility of the practitioner. This also applies to adherence to the boundaries of legally regulated medical and therapeutic practices. The fact that a book containing action proposals is freely available for sale does not imply that its application with clients or patients is permitted for everyone.

Hypnosis 1

You've realized that it's possible to let go of the fear in the darkness ... ... You've realized that it's possible to feel comfortable in the dark ... ... that's why you're here today ... ... You want to take a big step, to overcome the fear ... ... to feel comfortable even when it's dark outside ... ... You want to be able to sleep even in darkness ... ... Sleeping without light, that's your goal ... ... and this goal is achievable ... ... it really is achievable because with constructive and strong thoughts, you can accomplish more than you ever imagined ... ... It's important that your goal becomes a clear thought ... ... and that's what you'll achieve today ... ... in the trance you're now experiencing ... ... because in the state of trance, you're free from fear, you feel comfortable ... ... You're feeling calm and pleasantly relaxed right now ... ... and in this exact state, it's possible to form a constructive and helpful thought that changes everything ... ... to develop and firmly imprint a thought that truly helps you feel comfortable in the dark ... ... to let darkness become normal, because that's what it is ... ... completely normal ... ... You will achieve that today ... ... You'll achieve that especially well today ... ... Today is the first day of your new life ... ... Today is the first day of a life in freedom ... ... Freedom, even and especially in the dark ... ...

Darkness will become pleasant ... ... You know that darkness is part of the day's cycle, and at night, you want to feel comfortable ... ... After the sun has set, you want to feel safe even inside your home ... ... You're familiar with anxious thoughts that often troubled you ... ... and you know that thoughts can often intensify feelings ... ... So it's also possible to use thoughts of calm to make relaxation deeper ... ... You've experienced that just now, because you're in a state of pleasant relaxation ... ... even in a beautiful trance ... ... and in the same way, it's possible to use a helpful thought to strengthen your sense of security ... ... So you embrace the thought that tells you ... ... I feel safe and secure even in the darkness ... ... because this constructive thought can truly dissolve the fear ... ... and this thought helps you because it becomes the truth the more you think it or express it ... ...

Maybe you already know that your body always responds to your thoughts ... ... You thought of relaxation or heard the words of relaxation from me, and your body entered a wonderful trance ... ... because this state is good and because it feels good ... ... because you were inwardly ready for it and wanted it, you allowed the calm and relaxation ... ... and that's a good thing ... ... It's the same when your thought about darkness informs your body of relaxation ... ... You think ... ... I feel safe and secure even in the darkness ... ... and your body responds with these exact feelings ... ... because both can't happen at the same time ... ... You can't feel fear and security simultaneously ... ... You might think about fear now, but you feel calm and thus feel safe ... ... So as soon as your thought touches upon security and safety, you can't feel fear ... ... Your body responds with calmness ... ... and with a feeling of safety ... ...

This is how body and thoughts are interconnected ... ... and so are the feelings ... ... Everything within us influences each other ... ... Thoughts change the body, and the body changes the feelings ... ... Your helpful thought helps your body to relax ... ... more than that, your thought compels your body to calm down ... ... it can't be any other way ... ... as soon as you actively and consciously think ... ... I feel safe and secure even in the darkness ... ... your body automatically and immediately responds with relaxation … … and in doing so, your feelings relax too … … your mood improves, and your emotions become pleasant … … Fear then fades away, becomes impossible … … with a relaxed body, you can't feel fear … … a relaxed body always ensures a relaxed feeling … … and it's your thoughts that control your body … … only your thoughts … … Your thoughts can command your body to calm down, and that's exactly what you're doing … … it works now and every day … … especially, you can calm your body at night when it's dark … …

So now, and even in your waking life, you can be active and drive away any fear … … and replace the previous fear with feelings of calm and composure … … even a sense of safety … … a sense of security … … You face the darkness … … you can even sleep without light … … Yes, you can do it … … You can really do it … … Sleeping without light is now possible for you … … Sleeping without light is now natural for you because only your thoughts control your feelings … … So you consciously and deliberately think when turning off the light … … I feel safe and secure even in the darkness … … and immediately your body enters a state of calm … …

and you feel good in the dark ... ... you really feel good in the dark ... ...

You can be proud of yourself now ... ... proud because you've done it ... ... You've changed your feelings and reactions ... ... You've deeply anchored the new thought within you ... ... You've impressed it so deeply that it has become stronger than any possible thought of fear ... ... I feel safe and secure even in the darkness ... ... has become the strongest thought regarding darkness ... ... because you've embraced it in trance ... ... in a state of calm ... ... In the past, you used to think about darkness with fear, but today, you've changed darkness in a state of calm ... ... That's much easier ... ... and that's why you can now experience darkness and stay calm ... ... experience darkness and remain calm ... ... Sleeping without light is now possible ... ... Sleeping without light is now even more pleasant ... ... Sleeping without light ... ... Yes, sleeping without light ... ...

Hypnosis 2

You want to turn darkness into something different today … … You want to do something to experience darkness as normal, simply neutral … … or even pleasant … … You commit yourself to this goal and focus on it … … and that's why you'll succeed today in changing darkness … … first neutralizing it and then charging it positively … … Today, you'll achieve more than you thought possible … … much more than you thought … … Your possibilities today are enormous, so today you'll take two big steps … … Neutralizing darkness and then feeling good in the dark … … These are two big steps, and you're taking them in one go … … in a single session … … Today is your day because you're letting go of fear and building security … … Today is truly your special day … … because you're letting go of fear and building security … … Today is even the best day in a long, long time, because you're letting go of fear and building security … … You can do it … … You really can … … You'll do it faster and better than you can imagine … …

First, you reflect on your own competence, your abilities ... ... You remember that you've successfully faced many things in life and were always the one who had to rise to the occasion ... ... and that you succeeded ... ... You've always taken on life's challenges and overcome them ... ... Often it was your own ability to endure and to persevere in difficult situations that finally helped you to solve the challenges and problems on your path ... ... That's how it is today too ... ... today, you're successful from within ... ... You have the potential within you ... ... you're truly capable of leaving fear behind ... ... ending it today and then dealing with darkness in a relaxed way ... ... and today more than ever, you can tap into your potential ... ... unleash your deep inner competence and become aware of your strength and confidence ... ... so today, your inner strength and confidence replace the former fear ... ... and darkness is filled with your strength, with your power ... ... Darkness is filled with your competence ... ... You, very strong in the dark ... ...

First, we dispel the fear ... ... that's also possible with your potential ... ... with the abilities to overcome and let go, which have helped you in the past to master life's challenges

… … Deep inside, you now feel true relaxation, and relaxation also means composure … … Composure that helps you to now view darkness calmly … … Now, in this very moment, darkness is neutral … … because you feel good and it's dark inside you … … with closed eyes, it's dark, but you feel good … … Darkness is now neutral … … Darkness is more ordinary than before … … much more ordinary … … Darkness is completely ordinary now and doesn't matter at all … … and now you let go of thoughts of fear, you just let them go … … you focus strongly on letting go of fear because you don't need it and you don't feel it … … Darkness is okay now … … Now you even let go of the memory of fear thoughts, so they can't resurface … … Now, in this moment, you let go of everything connected to fear … … Fear thoughts leave now … … Fear thoughts really leave now, they truly disappear … … Fear thoughts really disappear now and forever … … and darkness is truly okay … …

Think of something beautiful … … a pleasant memory or a beautiful fantasy … … Now you're filled with positive and beautiful thoughts … … Now you're more and more flooded with beautiful thoughts … … Thoughts that are so beautiful they even reach into the darkness ... ... beautiful thoughts with light ... ... beautiful thoughts with darkness ... ... The most beautiful thoughts you can imagine flood you because now it's all about beautiful thoughts ... ... Now it's only the beautiful thoughts that matter, creating a new connection ... ... Imagine the most beautiful thing you have ... ... the most beautiful memory ... ... the most beautiful moment ... ... or the best fantasy you can have ... ... imagine it ... ... and with this beautiful thought, a new connection is made ... ... beautiful darkness, yes, yes, beautiful darkness ... ... beautiful darkness, yes, yes, beautiful darkness ... ...

In this moment, darkness changes, becomes beautiful ... ... because all the words you hear sink deep within you and stay there ... ... You succeed really well in making darkness pleasant and soon even enjoying it because you can sleep better in the dark ... ... Today, darkness becomes truly beautiful and good ... ... Darkness becomes truly beautiful and good ... ... You can be proud of yourself ... ... You can really be very proud of yourself because every change comes from within you ... ... from your inner self ... ... from your own strength ... ... You're doing really well ... ... really well, because you've truly succeeded in making darkness good … … You've succeeded … … You've succeeded … …

Two big steps are completed … … You've taken the fear out of the darkness and then even made it positive and pleasant … … You've done it … … You'll now experience darkness as completely okay … … as pleasant at night when you want to sleep … … You've really succeeded in making darkness something good … … into beautiful normality … … Darkness as beautiful normality … … So then, hold on to the feeling of success because it's your feeling … … You are successful … … You are truly successful and have managed to let go of fear and embrace darkness … … to accept it as normal and even helpful … …

Hypnosis 3

You've decided to dissolve the fear ... ... to dissolve and make the fear disappear ... ... You know the fear you often had ... ... fear in the dark and perhaps also anticipatory fear of the next darkness ... ... Let's call this fear and everything connected to it simply the fear of darkness ... ... There may be many reasons for it or many connections to the fear of darkness ... ... But when we talk about your fear of darkness now, we're talking about all the connections and associations of this feeling ... ... and all feelings are in our thoughts, but also in our body, because our body stores all feelings ... ... So, today you can use your body's perception and feeling to dissolve the fear of darkness ... ... That's possible ... ... That's really possible and it's happening today ... ... it's happening today ... ...

All the feelings we have also show up in our body because body and emotions are closely connected ... ... Pleasant feelings make the body relax and feel good ... ... they relieve tension and stress and even reduce pain ... ... or dissolve it ... ... and fear also expresses itself in our body ... ... causes muscle tension ... ... changes our breathing and our heartbeat ... ... You know this, you know the anxious tension ... ... so perhaps physical relaxation could already help dissolve the fear ... ... That's possible, and it's even quite easy to reduce fear through physical relaxation ... ... but there's more, and you want more ... ... You want to let go of the fear of darkness ... ... You want to let go of the fear of and in the darkness once and for all ... ... so you want more than just physical relaxation ... ... much more ... ... and there's more ... ... because there are also causes of fear ... ... background reasons for fear ... ... maybe you know them and know why you've often been so afraid in the dark or of the darkness ... ... or at least you know part of it ... ... But it doesn't really matter so much to know why it was often there or where this fear of darkness exactly came from ... ... It's more important and absolutely sufficient to know and recognize that every feeling, with all its entanglements, is stored in the body ... ... Fear doesn't just show up in physical reactions; it's stored in your body with all its causes, background reasons, and connections ... ... This fear is stored in your body ... ... and finding it is easier than you think ... ... You'll find it today ... ...

… … In your mind and in your feeling, scan your body from head to toe and find a spot that feels somehow different … … why it feels that way doesn't matter; what's important is finding a spot that stands out to you now … … maybe because you feel some pressure there or a slight pain … … a tension or some feeling that draws your attention … … There's a spot that stands out to you … … and even if it doesn't feel that way, it's there … … just pay attention to which part of your body comes to mind now … … which spot or body part immediately comes to your mind … … right now … … wherever that spot may be … … wherever … … If you're not sure, just pick one because you will choose the right one … … for sure … … That's where the fear is … … that's where the fear of darkness is now going … … that's where everything connected to your fear is gathering now … … All the information about your fear of darkness is going to this spot … … wherever it may be … … All the reasons stored in your body, all the connections your cells have stored, are going to this one spot … … good … … That's really good because your fear of darkness is gathering in this spot … … If you feel more pressure or tension there now, don't worry … … That's good because everything connected to your fear of darkness is indeed gathering there … … and that's important now … … it's really important now … … to have everything in one place, everything gathered in one spot … … your body can do that … … your body is doing that for you … … it's always done that with signals of tension, sometimes even with pain, but we don't always understand it … … we can't always recognize it, but now you recognize it because now you're gathering everything fearful … … gathering the fear of darkness in one place in your body … … and now the resolution begins … …

… … Focus completely on this spot in your body, which will feel better in a few moments … … better than ever before … … Direct your attention to this spot … … direct all your mindfulness to this spot and imagine a small light beginning to shine there … … in your body … … a light in your body, exactly where your fear of darkness is gathered … … The light becomes brighter … … with every breath, the light in your body becomes brighter and gradually dissolves the fear of darkness … … Imagine the light, which can dissolve the fear, becoming brighter and brighter … … brighter and brighter with every breath … … brighter and brighter with every breath … … and the fear of darkness dissolves … …

the fear of darkness dissolves ... ... You feel it because you feel this spot in your body becoming more and more relaxed ... ... With the image of the light there, which becomes ever brighter, the connections of fear dissolve from your body, and with that, the fear disappears ... ... because body and feeling are connected ... ... The light becomes brighter and brighter, and the fear of darkness disappears ... ... Fear dissolves ... ... Fear really dissolves ... ... Your body dissolves the fear in the light ... ...

Keep breathing calmly and evenly and trust that with every breath your body will continue to dissolve the fear of darkness and make it disappear ... ... even and especially when you're awake again because then your subconscious has the time and opportunity to keep dissolving the fear ... ... to flood your body with light and truly make the fear of darkness disappear ... ... Light or dark ... ... Only one is possible ... ... and you'll be flooded with light ... ... flooded with light ... ...

Hypnosis 4

You want to erase the fear in the darkness today ... ... That's possible because it's a feeling that was once part of you but now has truly outlived its usefulness ... ... You don't need this fear anymore ... ... it's a remnant from a long-past time ... ... it somehow got stuck, but now it's time to dissolve it ... ... and finally let your beautiful feelings be present again ... ... to connect beautiful feelings with darkness and with the night because the times of threats or fright are over ... ... Darkness is okay again ... ... You can use a strong thought, a thought that makes darkness normal ...

Imagine you're sleeping deeply ... ... It's night, and you've fallen asleep peacefully and are dreaming a beautiful dream ... ... maybe a vacation memory, or you're dreaming of an event, an experience that was truly wonderful ... ... and with the images in the dream, the old, beautiful feelings resurface ... ... maybe you know that we only dream of feelings ... ... and the dream images our subconscious produces are then images that match our feelings during sleep ... ... So you're dreaming beautiful images because you have beautiful feelings inside you … … Maybe you fall asleep with the light on because you feel safer that way … … or you often sleep without light but then transition to sleep somewhat uneasily … … but now you're sleeping and dreaming beautifully … … Your thoughts are becoming quieter and more tired … … so it's more and more the beautiful images that simply appear … … that are simply there and keep letting you feel pleasant feelings … … You just let yourself drift in the beautiful dream, which might be a very bright dream with a lot of light … …

Then, slowly, you wake up, and it's the middle of the night … … You wake up with the pleasant feelings of the dream … … You dreamed so beautifully that you wake up with a very good feeling … … still feeling comfortable and sleepily realizing that it's dark in your bedroom … … but the pleasant feeling from the dream is so strong that you feel comfortable even in the darkness of your bedroom … … You turn on a light and see a writing on the wall … … You can see it clearly because it's your thought written there … … On the wall, it reads … …

Darkness helps me focus on my feelings. In the dark, I feel connected with myself.

... [Read the affirmation slowly and a bit louder than the previous text, to emphasize it slightly. Then pause for about 30 seconds before continuing to read.] ...

Then you think about how it gets dark when we close our eyes ... ... and in the darkness of closed eyes, good sleep is also born, with beautiful and pleasant dreams ... ... with beautiful and pleasant feelings deep inside you ... ... So, you let the words you read on the wall resonate within you ... ... let them become a feeling deep inside you ... ... and this feeling within you gives you beautiful dreams once again ... ... Important words become inner beliefs ... ... deep convictions within you ... ... and the words you read on the bedroom wall become a very deep belief within you ... ... Now ... ... your deep conviction, the conviction of your feelings ... ... Now ... ... You fall asleep again, and your beautiful dreams become even more beautiful ... ... It is this thought, this formula, that makes your dreams so beautiful ... ... that makes falling asleep in the dark so easy ... ... It is this affirmation that you can think or say again and again ... ... It is this belief that you can repeat over and over again ... ... that becomes your mantra ... ... your inner wisdom ... ...

the security ... ... the firm belief that helps you to experience darkness naturally and to feel safe in the dark ... ...

These special words you heard from me and read on the bedroom wall resonate deeply within you, and you hear them once more ... ...

Darkness helps me focus on my feelings. In the dark, I feel connected with myself.

... [Read the affirmation slowly and a bit louder than the previous text, to emphasize it slightly. Then pause for about 30 seconds before continuing to read.] ...

... ... This is really good because these wise words unfold deeply within you and make darkness something helpful ... ... These words unfold the potential and beauty of darkness at night because your beautiful feelings awaken with the darkness ... ...

Your affirmation leads you to recognize darkness more and more as a helper and feel that darkness truly helps you focus on your beautiful feelings ... ... to feel your feelings because all the feelings you can feel and embrace help you to feel free ... ... and the feeling of freedom leads to the feeling of security ... ... and you can experience darkness naturally ... ... very naturally ... ... Every day, you can repeat this affirmation in a quiet moment with your eyes closed ... ... You can say it out loud or whisper it, however you like ... ... and make it even stronger ...

Hypnosis 5

You want to let go of the fear in the dark today … … because this fear has become a disturbing and burdensome feeling … … But you want to be carefree; you want to feel free … … and today, this liberation is possible … … Today, you can honor the fear as an important feeling because it was important … … It showed you that it was time to take care of yourself … … and that's exactly what you're doing because that's why you're here … … and because you're now taking care of yourself and your feelings, you can say goodbye to the fear today … … In a few moments, you can speak with your deepest self and honor the fear and, at the same time, let it go … … That's how you'll succeed today in changing the darkness in your feelings … … Your subconscious is supporting you because it hears and understands every word I say because it becomes your own word … … It is you who says … …

… … I feel safe even in the dark … … because I'm aware that I am strong and grown-up … …

... ... I feel safe even in the dark ... ... because I'm aware that fearful thoughts belong to the past ... ...

... ... I feel safe even in the dark ... ... because I'm aware that my home is as safe at night as it is during the day in the light ... ...

... ... I feel safe even in the dark ... ... because I'm aware that darkness is part of the night just as light is part of the day ... ...

... ... It's always bright inside me ... ... Deep inside me, it's always bright ... ...

... ... I focus on the naturalness of darkness ... ... because that helps me to accept darkness as natural ... ...

... ... I focus on the naturalness of darkness ... ... because darkness can also help me find restful sleep ... ...

... ... I focus on the naturalness of darkness ... ... because I know that my constructive thoughts help me accept darkness ... ...

... ... I focus on the naturalness of darkness ... ... because this also allows me to naturally deal with day and night ... ... with light and dark ... ...

… … It's always bright inside me … … Deep inside me, it's always bright … …

… … Darkness helps my body to feel comfortable in a natural rhythm … … that's why my body surely looks forward to the darkness of night … …

… … Darkness helps my body to feel comfortable in a natural rhythm … … that's why my body can regenerate best in the dark … …

… … Darkness helps my body to feel comfortable in a natural rhythm … … that's why I'll soon feel that I'm physically more vital and healthier … …

… … Darkness helps my body to feel comfortable in a natural rhythm … … that's why my whole being adjusts to accepting darkness … …

… … It's always bright inside me … … Deep inside me, it's always bright … …

… … I honor my previous fear as an important feeling … … because I've understood that accepting my feelings can set me free … …

... ... I honor my previous fear as an important feeling ... ... because I've understood that I don't have to fight against myself, but I can be connected to myself with self-love ... ...

... ... I honor my previous fear as an important feeling ... ... because I've understood that this feeling ensured I'm now taking care of myself ... ...

... ... I honor my previous fear as an important feeling ... ... because I've understood that I can finally say goodbye to it by acknowledging it ... ...

... ... It's always bright inside me ... ... Deep inside me, it's always bright ... ...

... ... From now on, I face the darkness at night ... ... and that's why I feel safe and secure ... ...

... ... From now on, I face the darkness at night ... ... and that's why I sleep without light and feel good doing it ... ...

... ... From now on, I face the darkness at night ... ... and that's why feelings of security and calm replace the former fear ... ...

... ... From now on, I face the darkness at night ... ... and that's why darkness truly becomes my ally ... ...

… … It's always bright inside me … … Deep inside me, it's always bright … … [30 seconds of silence] … …

The most important thing is done … … You've taken the fear out of the darkness and prepared yourself to say goodbye to it … … You honored it today and with that, you let it go, you released it … … so now you can do this every day … … You're free from fear, and as soon as it could arise, you say goodbye to it because now darkness is normal … … Now darkness at night is part of inner peace and restful sleep … … and it's always bright inside you … … deep inside you, it's always bright … …

Hypnosis 6

Your goal is to experience darkness better ... ... to look forward to the darkness of night with free thoughts and just let it happen ... ... You want to feel good again at night, to live naturally and normally with darkness ... ... For that, you're taking a special path today ... ... You're turning today to a special instance that can help you ... ... You're turning to someone you can believe in because you're sure you'll find help there ... ... maybe to your subconscious because you believe in inner power ... ... or you can better speak with an inner helper because you know that you're speaking with your strong inner parts, with a powerful part of yourself that can help ... ... Perhaps you also believe in God's help or the help of a guardian angel; then you can ask for their help ... ... say a prayer in trance ... ... In trance, all the connections you need are accessible, and all thoughts unfold well and constructively ... ... So, speak to the instance you can best believe in, with the following words, which are your own words ... ...

Dear subconscious / Dear inner helper / Dear guardian angel ... ... I need support in finding peace in the darkness ... ... Peace and a free feeling, so I can be alone in the dark and sleep well at night ... ... I ask for your support on this path ... ... Support on the path to finding peace within myself again and to experience darkness naturally ... ... Perhaps you can first help me to better endure the darkness ... ... To endure it even when I feel fear arising, and to give me the security that I can remain calm despite fear ... ... this will make it easier for me to deal with the darkness and take the next step ... ... after I can better endure darkness and even the rising thoughts of fear than before ... ...

Dear subconscious / Dear inner helper / Dear guardian angel ... ... I ask for your help in becoming freer in the dark with each passing day ... ... to feel more and more that the fear is shrinking and disappearing with each passing day ... ... until finally, the fear is completely gone, and I can feel completely free again, especially in the dark ... ... with your help, I can do this ... ... with your help, I'll manage this ... ... Dear subconscious / Dear inner helper / Dear guardian angel ... ... I trust your help and guidance, and I know that with your help and guidance, I will overcome the fear ... ... once and for all ... ...

Dear subconscious / Dear inner helper / Dear guardian angel ... ... I know that it's often unseen feelings that later burden us as fear ... ... I'm aware that there have been things in my life that were left behind, things I need to catch up on ... ... I know that I didn't always have the strength and time to take care of myself ... ... I also know and accept with your help that this wasn't my fault, that it happened without me being able to foresee it ... ... Dear subconscious / Dear inner helper / Dear guardian angel ... ... I ask for your support in truly experiencing myself as innocent and being patient with myself, even when the release from fear doesn't happen as quickly as I'd like ... ... so that in the end, I do succeed ... ... with your help and guidance ... ...

Dear subconscious / Dear inner helper / Dear guardian angel ... ... I want to start today by being patient and empathetic with myself ... ... I embrace myself internally with love ... ... I bring as much self-love as possible ... ... and I ask for help in truly being able to accept myself ... ... to truly love myself ... ... I know it's possible, and I know I can do it ... ... with your help and guidance, I'll succeed even faster and more clearly in accepting myself with love … … in truly accepting myself with love … … Dear subconscious / Dear inner helper / Dear guardian angel … … I trust your help and thank you for the guidance and support on my path to liberation … …

Now, take a rest … … Give yourself a moment to pause and let the words you've heard sink in … … Trust that a part of you has understood these words as your own and has spoken them with me … … and another part of you has listened as a helping instance and will help you achieve your goal … … and the instance you've chosen deep within you, the one you've spoken to, will also help you … … whoever it may be … …

Hypnosis 7

Darkness should be easier today … … it should be easier to experience darkness with a good feeling … … You used to be able to do this because there was a time when you didn't even think about being afraid in the dark … … No one brings this fear into the world … … It was events and experiences that led to the fear in or of the darkness … … but that's over … … it's long ago, and today it no longer fits … … Today, you're safe in the darkness and want to feel safe … … just as it used to be, however long ago that may be … … You'll find that former self-confidence today because it's still within you … … You can awaken it today … … and become self-confident again … … so self-confident that you can experience darkness as ordinary … …

Remember the time before the fear … … there was a time before the fear because no one is born with such fear … … So, you can now return to that time … … maybe you know when that was … … Perhaps you can't remember exactly when the fear of and in the dark began … … it may have been a gradual process … … but if you think back far enough, you'll find a time when you didn't have this fear … … Think back five years, how was it then? … … Feel whether you could be in the dark without fear at that time … … and now go back another five years … … Feel once more how it was then, ten years ago … … maybe you've already reached a time without fear … … but on your journey through time in your mind, you can go back further … … many years … … So, go even further back if it helps you, and find a time when you naturally dealt with darkness … … a time when you knew that everything was okay even in the dark because back then everything was okay … … whenever that was … … You don't need to know exactly how old you were then … … it's enough to imagine and intend to find that time … … and in your deep feeling, you'll find the memory of that fear-free time … … even if it was so far back that you were still in the womb, not yet born … … no one feels fear in the womb … … there is pure security … … even this memory is stored in your inner self … … as a feeling that you now rediscover … … as a deep and clear memory within you … …

Now, be mindful and feel your deep emotion … … Pay attention to your body's feeling, signaling you calmness and composure … … safety and security … … and pay attention to your mood … … to the feeling of calm … … Fear is impossible now because you are inwardly and outwardly calm … … Now, only calm is possible and a good feeling … … Now, even the thought of darkness is bearable and lets you remain calm … … That's how it was back then too … … that's how it was before the fear, and you're in that time now … … in the time before the fear … … that's how it was, and that's how it can be again … … Back then, you had no fear … … back then, you had exactly this good feeling that you're feeling now … … that's why you could sleep well in the dark … … that's why it didn't bother you at all when it got dark outside, and you were still awake … … or you were alone … … Darkness was outside, but it was harmless … … completely harmless … … You're back in that earlier time in your imagination, before the fear … … in that earlier time with all its good feelings … … and these good feelings are now awakening again within you … … because now your subconscious remembers and knows that you need these old feelings now … … these good feelings … … and your body also remembers how it was … … because the body stores all feelings in its cells … … Now your entire being truly remembers how to feel strong and self-confident even in darkness ... ... You remember deep within how to feel your own confidence and security even and especially in the dark ... ... and to use your confidence and security at that moment ... ... and to feel good in the darkness ... ... You remember ... ... That's how it was back then ... ... That's how it is now because you are now internally in that time ... ... because you are in that strong time ... ... in your feeling, you are there ... ... truly ...

And with this feeling, you move forward internally ... ... just as your path led you back, you now move forward into the future ... ... So, go ahead ... ... year by year ... ... Imagine moving forward with these good feelings from back then, which you are now truly feeling, into the future ... ... beyond today, you go forward with all your good feelings ... ... with your self-confidence ... ... with your naturalness and completely free of any conceivable fear ... ... with composure and ease, you move forward ... ... arriving from the present into a near future ... ... perhaps a few weeks or months ahead, and feel within yourself ... ... you still feel the good feelings from back then because you've revived them ... ... You are in the future and feel strong and free like before ... ... unburdened and free like before ... ... the self-confidence and freedom from before, especially in the future ... ... and fear of darkness has disappeared ... ... You don't feel it now ... ... and now you are in the future ... ... without the fear ...

And so you can now return with your good feelings ... ... return to the present only with good feelings ... ... return to the present day ... ... completely without fear because now there is only self-confidence ... ... Self-confidence, especially in the dark, because that's when you need it most ... ... In a few moments, you will wake up again and bring the former strength with you, the self-confidence ... ... Fear remains only in memory ... ... You wake up with self-confidence and composure and bring them into your everyday life ... ... Self-confidence and composure you take with you into the darkness ... ... to feel only self-confidence and composure, especially in the dark ... ...

Hypnosis 8

+++ Instructions for Implementation +++

This hypnosis uses ideomotor response. Ideomotor response refers to the phenomenon that our body follows our feelings and thoughts with movements. In everyday life, this following shows as body posture, muscle tension, and movement patterns that naturally change with mood and thoughts. In trance, ideomotor signals can be used to obtain information that the client cannot actively communicate. For example, the subconscious can answer questions with a prearranged finger signal. Of course, ideomotor responses can also be used suggestively, such as with arm levitations and catalepsy. An ideomotor approach strengthens trust in hypnosis and in one's ability to change, thereby promoting therapy.

+++ End of Instructions +++

Today, you want to do something to finally let go of your fear in and of the darkness ... ... so you can deal with darkness naturally because you experience and recognize darkness as a natural occurrence ... ... and that's especially possible in cooperation with your subconscious ... ... because in hypnosis, in the deep relaxation you can feel now, you can actually cooperate with the subconscious ... ... and the best part is that your subconscious can give you a noticeable and visible response ... ... It can and will confirm and prove to you that the two of you are really working successfully together and that you are truly letting go of the old fear of and in the dark ... ... I will help you with this ... ... Maybe you're wondering how this works and how your subconscious can give you a visible and noticeable sign ... ... a sign of successful cooperation ... ... a sign of successful cooperation ... ... maybe you already know this ... ... whatever the case, you're about to experience it ... ...

New things can always occur and become reality when we succeed in building a really clear picture of what we want to achieve ... ... our target visualization is the key to success ... ... because a constructive and clear target visualization embeds itself so deeply that the new emerges in our lives from it ... ... The new thing in your life should be freedom ... ... Freedom from fear ... ... Freedom to feel good ... ...

Freedom to be relaxed … … Freedom in the dark … … true freedom in the dark … … So, imagine what that should be like … … Imagine yourself with a good feeling in the darkness … … no matter how new this picture may be, in trance, you can imagine it … … however unusual this idea may still be, however unfamiliar it may still be … … in your imagination, you are free in the dark … … free in the dark … … as free and relaxed as you feel now, or even freer … … even better than now … … Imagine, for example, that you're at home, alone, but you feel good … … It's dark outside, but you feel good … … Imagine you're going to bed, lying down, but you feel good … … really good … … It's dark; the light is off, but you feel good … … You really feel good … … You can imagine it, at least as a fantasy, as an idea of how it should be … … That works very well … … because that's how it should be … … You want to be able to feel good in the dark, just sleep peacefully … … free from fear … … free with a good feeling … … free with relaxation … … free in the dark … … free in the dark … … Imagine it so it can become reality … … The more clearly you imagine it, the faster it becomes reality … … good …

Hold on to this image of freedom now ... ... because this image should shape the darkness ... ... Your subconscious will help you with this ... ... The more you can hold on to this image and see it before your mind's eye, the faster your subconscious can also make this vision your new reality ... ... true freedom in the dark ... ... and as soon as your subconscious has done this, and it will do it, one of your right-hand fingers will move clearly ... ... as a signal that this inner transformation has truly taken place ... ... Your subconscious will show you when it's done, when it has erased the fear and built freedom because only then will it move a finger ... ... only then, when it has made this the reality, will a finger of your right hand move ... ... Imagine the goal, as a picture ... ... as a visualization ... ... You are free in the dark, and your subconscious now makes that a reality, so that it can only be that way, that you are free in the dark and also feel free ... ... and as soon as the fear is erased and freedom built, a finger of your right hand moves clearly ... ... a finger of your right hand moves as a signal of freedom from fear ... ... It will happen as soon as your subconscious has erased the fear ... ...

[Try to be patient until a finger clearly moves because it will happen. Ideomotor signals are reliable signs. Here, we are working with a mix of suggestive prompting and ideomotor communication. When you repeatedly say ... a finger moves ... it has a suggestive effect, and the ideomotor response will occur sooner or later. By implying that this resolves fear and builds a pleasant feeling, a connection is made in the unconscious. The subconscious confirms by moving a signal finger that fear has been resolved. If it couldn't enable this, it wouldn't make sense to move a signal finger. However, if the movement happens "only" due to suggestions, it still serves as proof of effectiveness for the conscious mind, as this was the "agreement." If the conscious mind is convinced, the goal is almost achieved. Doubts? Then just try it and be amazed together with your client!]

Your subconscious has resolved the fear, you felt the signal, and I saw it ... ... and therefore, you will experience darkness much more freely and relaxed ... ... Your subconscious now gives you back control of your hand ... ... You have full control over your hand, over each finger ... ...

Move your hand and fingers, and check that your fingers are indeed fully under your conscious control ... ...

[Always make sure the client has their hands and fingers under conscious and active control again and can move them. Let them actively try. If it doesn't work, help with further suggestions ... Your fingers are completely relaxed now, very loose. Very, very loose are your fingers ... You can move them now ...]

Your subconscious has worked with you to resolve the fear ... ... With your visualization and concentration, you did your part, and your subconscious helped by resolving the fear deeply and clearly showed you by moving the signal finger that it had done so ... ... and you can rely on your subconscious ... ... It is reliable ... ... It confirmed that the fear is gone, so it is also gone ... ... truly gone ... ...

Hypnosis 9

+++ Instructions for Implementation +++

A self-hypnosis trigger is a signal that initiates the state of trance. With its help, even an inexperienced client can continue working with self-hypnosis at home. Of course, they can "only" work with simple suggestions they can easily remember and that we should prepare, or with simple visualizations. Triggered self-hypnosis is a very good tool to give the client a task to take home and support the therapy. This way, the time between appointments in the practice is not without therapy but is continued at home. Fully self-guided self-hypnosis, without a trigger, is also good to learn but requires much time and practice. Setting up the trigger is a relatively simple task and naturally relieves the client, whom I don't want to burden with training self-guided self-hypnosis. Contrary to all naysayers, I also claim here that it's really not a problem to teach a client simple triggered self-hypnosis. It's no more dangerous than meditation, autogenic training, or yoga. You survive those too unscathed at home. I've seen numerous patients in my practice who not only managed well with self-hypnosis but enjoyed it. And if a patient enjoys self-hypnosis, however simple the suggestion may look, then that is a very good support for compliance. Discuss the procedure once before hypnosis and give the client a short keyword list of the steps of self-hypnosis so they have a little guide.

+++ End of Instructions +++

Today, I'll show you how self-hypnosis works because with self-hypnosis, you can help yourself quickly let go of fear ... ... even when you're at home ... ... when you're all alone ... ... especially then, and for that, you need self-hypnosis ... ... You can use it over and over again, three times a day if you want ... ... twice in broad daylight and once as soon as it gets dark ... ... so you can keep letting go of the fear or ensure it doesn't arise again ... ... Self-hypnosis is simple and really safe ... ... I'll show you how it works and help you set up a trigger now that will help you ... ... a trigger is like a switch that can turn on the trance for you ... ... when you activate it, you slowly but surely go into trance ... ... just as your trance feels now, so will the self-hypnosis feel ... ...

Now, concentrate entirely on the relaxation you feel ... ... That's trance ... ... You know it well and experience it here ... ... a completely natural state that you can create for yourself at home ... ... All you need is a trigger, a little help ... ... You have it with you; it's the ball of your left thumb ... ... Now, grasp the ball of your left thumb with your right hand and massage it with light pressure using your right thumb ... ...

[Please discuss and demonstrate this before hypnosis, so it works well. No special technique is required, just let them massage the thumb ball] ... ...

This is the signal for your body to go into trance ... ... just like now ... ... As soon as you lie down, close your eyes, and massage your thumb ball, you'll go into trance, into the same state of relaxation as now ... ... Your body will store it this way for you ... ... good ... ... already done ... ... As soon as you massage your thumb ball with your eyes closed, you'll go into trance ... ... very simple ...

Then, you let your trance go even deeper by quietly saying ten times ... ... truly deep peace ... ... As you do this, you count to ten, which is very simple and makes the trance even more stable ... ... You just whisper ... ... once truly deep peace … … twice truly deep peace … … three times truly deep peace … … and so on … … until you finally reach ten and whisper … … ten times truly deep peace … … and in doing so, you'll naturally sink into a beautiful trance … … part of you stays awake and guides your self-hypnosis … … another part goes into deep trance …

[For deepening and the main part, I recommend counting with the suggestions … once … twice, etc. This has the advantage that the client is not distracted by wondering how many times they've repeated the suggestion. It doesn't really matter if they don't hit exactly ten repetitions; in trance, this helps them stay on track. You can, of course, speak all ten repetitions aloud in the teachings. After all, you're also working suggestively in this hypnosis, so it's not just a self-hypnosis training but hypnosis.]

Then comes the part where you can change the darkness … … above all, you can change your way of dealing with darkness by using a short and very helpful suggestion … … You just whisper it ten times … … Ten times you say … … I am and remain calm, even in the dark … … Again, you count … … You say … … I am and remain calm, even once in the dark … … I am and remain calm, even twice in the dark … …

I am and remain calm, even three times in the dark ... ... until you finally say ... ... I am and remain calm, even ten times in the dark ... ... and then you just breathe calmly in and out a few times and make sure you feel really good ...

To wake up again, to return from trance, imagine a cold wind blowing ... ... Imagine you're standing in a cold wind, and then you say ... ... Enough now, I'm waking up ... ... and then you count loudly and clearly to three and open your eyes ... ... You can do this, it's easy ... ... so once again ... ... To wake up, imagine you're standing in a cold wind, and then you say ... ... Enough now, I'm waking up – One – Two – Three ... ... and then you're fully awake and open your eyes ... ... very simple ...

You now know how it works ... ... You can start working with your self-hypnosis right away and keep changing the darkness until you soon feel completely comfortable in the dark ... ... Your subconscious has learned for you to go into trance with your thumb trigger ... ... simply by initiating the trance with your thumb, which you then deepen with the words ... truly deep peace ... ... Then follows your suggestion ... I am and remain calm, even in the dark ... and then you imagine a cold wind and say aloud and clearly ... Enough now, I'm waking up – One – Two – Three ... ... Then you open your eyes and are fully awake ...

Hypnosis 10

We're taking a journey together today … … a journey that's only possible because you can dive deep into your imagination … … because you have access to your creativity and can find the way inward … … In your dreams, you can think about anything that's possible or seemingly impossible … … But often, much more is possible than we think because imagination and reality are very close together, so close that we sometimes can't properly distinguish between them … … and don't need to, because any daydream can become reality if the right time for it comes … … Maybe the right time is today … … right now, at this very moment … … Maybe now is the right moment to overcome the fear in and of the darkness … … so you focus your attention and mindfulness on the center of your body, where your gut feeling resides … … and you imagine that you could sink with your entire awareness into this point … … deeper and deeper into yourself, to fully be in your feeling … … to now arrive in the land of your dreams …

Imagine you're standing in the middle of a beautiful old street, looking directly at a beautiful house … … a house with tall windows and doors, an old house that looks like it grew naturally in this landscape … … Walk towards the house … … it's your inner house … … It's built strong and secure … … has withstood rough times and still stands firm like a rock in the storm … … The house is like you … … deep inside, unshakeable and stable because disturbances usually only come from the outside … … and then in our thoughts … … but from the perspective of our feelings, thoughts are also outside … … far outside even … … and much deeper lie the feelings … … much deeper lies the land of dreams … … Open the door of the house … … It opens very easily … … Step into your inner house …

… … In the entryway, you find wardrobes … … You can leave everything you don't need right now in them … … All thoughts, all worries, all feelings you can put down like a backpack and store in the wardrobes … … maybe there's a lot of baggage you need to leave here … … So, you put it down … … Then you walk further down the hallway of the house … … there are many doors here … … many rooms where you can find events and experiences from your life …

... and possibilities ... ... because there are always more possibilities and more options than we think ... ... we don't always recognize them ... ... but in the land of dreams, you always see more than in your waking life ... ... because that is far away ... ... You come to a door with a sign that says ... ... Room of Safety ... ... Open the door and go inside ... ... The room is empty ... ... It's meant to be your place of absolute safety ... ... your refuge ... ... maybe your panic room ... ... a room where nothing can happen to you, absolutely nothing ...

... ... Think about what you might need in this room of calm and safety ... ... Choose a piece of furniture that can give you comfort ... ... maybe a comfortable couch or an armchair ... ... or a cozy mattress with a fluffy blanket ... ... or whatever suits you best ... ... whatever can best help you feel secure ... ... Set up this piece of furniture and try it out ... ... Make yourself comfortable on it and let it work for you ... ... Feel how it actually already gives you a sense of safety ... ... Set up the room further ... ... Maybe you need a table, a few shelves, or other pieces of furniture that come to mind ... ... Choose everything so that you can feel comfortable ... ... and safe ... ... Now think about how you can protect yourself in this room ... ... Install a secure lock on the door and your window ... ... a lock that you can operate very easily ... ... that gives you absolute security so that nothing and no one can enter your room without your permission ...

... ... Now think of a way to communicate ... ... Maybe you want a secure phone so you can contact the outside without fear ... ... so you can remain anonymous if you wish ... ... Perhaps you'd prefer a radio or an internet connection ... ... with a webcam ... ... Decide for yourself what gives you the most security and how you want to reach out when you want to retreat to safety ... ... Decide for yourself how you want to communicate ... ... how you want to talk about your fear ... ... You can be in a safe place and still send messages ... ... So, decide who you want in your contact list ... ... Try out your communication methods now ... ... Imagine calling someone and talking to someone about your fear ... ... You know that nothing can happen to you in this safe place and that you can immediately distance yourself from it ... ... So only you decide how you communicate ...

... ... Now think about who you want to visit you in this safe place ... ... who is allowed access to your inner house to visit you, especially when you retreat deep into this house ...

... Arrange with this visitor a signal you'll give them so that they can enter your safe room ... ... Maybe someone should have a key whom you fully trust or the access code to your security lock on the door ... ... You'll also need some food in your safe room ... ... maybe a fridge or a microwave ... ... You can also set up a dumbwaiter where your meals will be delivered if you need to stay in your room longer ... ... Plan your room exactly the way it can be the safest retreat, the best hideout for you ... ... And then enjoy the peace and the feeling of security in your room ... ... Lock the door if you want and stay completely in this room ... ... Let it become the place of inner retreat ... ... You can go there whenever darkness scares you ...

Deep inside you, there's always a place of safety ... ... in the land of dreams ... ... and with just a thought, you're there when you want to be, and you feel truly safer ... ... Is that only possible in imagination? ... ... No, it's possible mainly in feelings ... ... because the land of dreams lies deep within you ... ... it's always been there ... ... I'm just telling you about it ... ...

All Titles in the Series

Volume 1: Smoking Cessation
Volume 2: Anxiety and Restlessness
Volume 3: Burnout
Volume 4: Reducing Overweight
Volume 5: Coping with the Past
Volume 6: Suicidal Thoughts and Attempts
Volume 7: Psycho-Oncology
Volume 8: Obsessions and Tics
Volume 9: Self-Confidence and Decision-Making
Volume 10: Grief Work
Volume 11: Psychosomatics
Volume 12: Chronic Pain
Volume 13: Depressive Thoughts
Volume 14: Panic Attacks
Volume 15: Domestic Violence, Victim Support
Volume 16: Post-Traumatic Stress
Volume 17: Exam Anxiety and Stage Fright
Volume 18: Anti-Violence Training, Offender Support
Volume 19: Addiction Tendencies
Volume 20: Social Phobia and Fear of Contact
Volume 21: Nail Biting
Volume 22: Self-Awareness and Self-Love
Volume 23: Teeth Grinding and Night Clenching
Volume 24: Feelings of Guilt
Volume 25: Fear in Crowds
Volume 26: Fear of Flying, Aviophobia
Volume 27: Fear in Enclosed Spaces, Claustrophobia
Volume 28: Tinnitus, Ear Noises
Volume 29: Fear of Heights
Volume 30: Neurodermatitis

Volume 31: Finding Inner Balance
Volume 32: Overcoming Loneliness
Volume 33: Fear of Illness, Hypochondria
Volume 34: Anticipatory Anxiety, Fear of Fear
Volume 35: Jealousy in Relationships
Volume 36: Driving Anxiety
Volume 37: New Start after Separation
Volume 38: Fear of Injections
Volume 39: Heart Anxiety Neurosis
Volume 40: Overcoming Resentment and Anger
Volume 41: Resolving Blockages and Positive Thinking
Volume 42: Stress Reduction, Stress Management
Volume 43: Body Relaxation
Volume 44: Deep Relaxation
Volume 45: Fear of the Dark
Volume 46: Falling Asleep and Staying Asleep
Volume 47: Compulsive Buying
Volume 48: Restless Legs Syndrome
Volume 49: Bulimia
Volume 50: Anorexia
Volume 51: Overcoming Nightmares
Volume 52: Imagined Deformity
Volume 53: Overcoming Distrust, Finding Trust
Volume 54: Processing Failures
Volume 55: Humiliation, Emotional Hurt
Volume 56: Distressing Compassion, Vicarious Suffering
Volume 57: Self-Forgiveness
Volume 58: Self-Awareness, Self-Confidence
Volume 59: Saying No
Volume 60: Assertiveness
Volume 61: Setting Boundaries and Self-Assertion
Volume 62: Decision-Making Ability

Volume 63: Success Orientation
Volume 64: Ruminating, Circular Thinking
Volume 65: Accepting Pregnancy
Volume 66: Birth Preparation
Volume 67: Spiritual Opening
Volume 68: Joy of Life and Inner Lightness
Volume 69: Patience and Inner Peace
Volume 70: Fibromyalgia and Rheumatism
Volume 71: Irritable Bowel Syndrome, Crohn's Disease
Volume 72: Fear of Nausea, Emetophobia
Volume 73: Stuttering and Cluttering, Speech Flow Disorders
Volume 74: Concentration and Knowledge Anchoring
Volume 75: Vitality and Spontaneity
Volume 76: Searching for Meaning and Finding Goals
Volume 77: Life Crises, Life Events
Volume 78: Workaholism, Goal Obsession
Volume 79: Helper Syndrome, Helpless Helpers
Volume 80: Medication Abuse
Volume 81: Gambling Addiction
Volume 82: Internet Addiction, Smartphone Addiction
Volume 83: Hoarding Disorder, Compulsive Collecting
Volume 84: Conspiracy Thoughts, Overvalued Ideas
Volume 85: Fear of Operations and Treatments
Volume 86: Fear of Aging
Volume 87: Travel Anxiety
Volume 88: Anxiety When Urinating, Paruresis
Volume 89: Fear of Intimacy and Togetherness
Volume 90: Fear of Blushing
Volume 91: Coming Out in Homosexuality
Volume 92: Charisma Training
Volume 93: Migraines and Chronic Headaches
Volume 94: Overcoming Allergies, Bronchial Asthma

Volume 95: Normalizing Blood Pressure
Volume 96: Compulsive Perfectionism
Volume 97: Sports Hypnosis, Motivation
Volume 98: Sports Hypnosis, Performance Enhancement
Volume 99: Determination and Focus
Volume 100: Encountering the Inner Child
Volume 101: Cravings, Binge Eating
Volume 102: Stimulating Metabolism
Volume 103: Bipolar Mood Swings
Volume 104: Borderline, Identity Crises
Volume 105: Hypomania, Euphoria, Mania
Volume 106: Restlessness, Agitation
Volume 107: Nervous Breakdown
Volume 108: Adjustment Disorders
Volume 109: Self-Alienation, Depersonalization
Volume 110: Ending Self-Pity
Volume 111: Primary Gain of Illness
Volume 112: Secondary Gain of Illness
Volume 113: Bullying, Victim Support
Volume 114: Letting Go of Envy and Jealousy
Volume 115: Fear of Spiders, Arachnophobia
Volume 116: Fear of Dogs or Cats
Volume 117: Fear of Strangers, Xenophobia
Volume 118: Excessive Worries, Generalized Anxiety
Volume 119: Strengthening Sense of Responsibility
Volume 120: Unrequited Love, Heartache
Volume 121: Work-Life Balance
Volume 122: Letting Go of Unattainable Goals
Volume 123: Allowing and Accepting Help
Volume 124: Letting Go of Adult Children
Volume 125: Tourette Syndrome
Volume 126: Life Changes and New Starts

Volume 127: Accepting Life in a Wheelchair
Volume 128: Understanding and Overcoming Homesickness
Volume 129: Understanding and Overcoming Wanderlust
Volume 130: Dizziness, Meniere's Disease
Volume 131: Overcoming Aggression
Volume 132: Cutting and Self-Harm
Volume 133: Hair Pulling, Trichotillomania
Volume 134: Postpartum Depression
Volume 135: For Relatives of Dementia Patients
Volume 136: Self-Harm, Artificial Disorders
Volume 137: Activating Self-Healing Powers
Volume 138: Preventing Depression Relapse
Volume 139: Reactive Psychoses, Follow-Up
Volume 140: Obsessive Thoughts and Impulses
Volume 141: Compulsive Checking
Volume 142: Compulsive Counting, Symmetry Obsession
Volume 143: Compulsive Washing, Cleanliness Obsession
Volume 144: Compulsive Questioning
Volume 145: Dissociative Paralysis
Volume 146: Phantom Pain
Volume 147: Overcoming Complaining
Volume 148: Hay Fever, Pollen Allergy
Volume 149: Sexual Abuse, Victim Support
Volume 150: Standing Strong Against Sexism, #metoo
Volume 151: Binge Eating
Volume 152: Overcoming Thoughts of Revenge
Volume 153: Detachment from the Aggressor, Stockholm Syndrome
Volume 154: Courage to Separate
Volume 155: Chronic Fatigue, Exhaustion
Volume 156: Fear of the Future, Existential Anxiety
Volume 157: Excessive Worry About Children
Volume 158: Fear of Failure

Volume 159: Ending Distrust and Control
Volume 160: Dejection, Dysphoria
Volume 161: Boreout, Chronic Boredom
Volume 162: Bipolar Disorders, Relapse Prevention
Volume 163: Mania, Relapse Prevention
Volume 164: Nihilism, Feelings of Worthlessness
Volume 165: Thumb Sucking
Volume 166: Being Brave
Volume 167: Being Proud
Volume 168: Overcoming Shyness
Volume 169: Being Able to Delegate Responsibility
Volume 170: Being Able to Show Emotions
Volume 171: Letting Go of Guilt, Victim Support
Volume 172: Processing Guilt, Offender Support
Volume 173: Mood Swings, Cyclothymia
Volume 174: Lack of Drive, Vital Sadness
Volume 175: Hearing Voices with Reality Reference
Volume 176: Confident Communication
Volume 177: Standing Up for Oneself
Volume 178: Taking New Paths
Volume 179: Confident Job Application
Volume 180: No Longer Being Taken Advantage Of
Volume 181: End of Submissiveness
Volume 182: Depressive Numbness
Volume 183: Mood Drops, Affective Incontinence
Volume 184: Mood Instability
Volume 185: Somatoform Disorders
Volume 186: Stomach Ulcer, Psychosomatic
Volume 187: Accepting Amputation
Volume 188: Overcoming and Letting Go of Hatred
Volume 189: Ending Accusations
Volume 190: Allowing Tears, Being Able to Cry

Volume 191: Finding and Sorting Repressed Feelings
Volume 192: Somatoform Pain
Volume 193: Living Autonomously
Volume 194: Anhedonia, Joylessness
Volume 195: Persistent Sadness
Volume 196: Obesity, Food Addiction
Volume 197: Parents of Abused Children
Volume 198: Letting Go and Letting Be
Volume 199: Childhood Sexual Abuse
Volume 200: Fear of Loss

www.ingramcontent.com/pod-product-compliance
Lightning Source LLC
Chambersburg PA
CBHW031531210526
45464CB00012B/2633